# FIBROID

## Unveiling the truth about your treatment

**Dr. Prince Marvelous**

# TABLE OF CONTENTS

# Presentation

Discover the secret of Fibroid pain without surgery

What is a fibroid? Fibroids are growths made of smooth muscle cells and sinewy connective tissue that foster in the uterus. It is assessed that 70 to 80 percent of ladies will foster fibroids in the course of their life  in any case, not every person will foster side effects or require treatment.

The main trait of fibroids is that they're quite often harmless, or noncancerous. All things considered, a few fibroids start as disease however harmless fibroids can't become malignant growth.

Destructive fibroids are exceptionally interesting. On account of this reality, it's sensible for ladies without side effects to pick perception as opposed to treatment.

Concentrates on showing that fibroids develop at various rates, in any event, when a lady has multiple. They can go from the size of a pea to (sometimes) the size of a watermelon. Regardless of whether fibroids develop that enormous, we offer opportune and viable treatment to give help.

Uterine fibroids are the most well-known cancer of the regenerative lot.

Ladies who are approaching menopause are at the most serious gamble for fibroids.

Fibroids are most frequently found during a routine pelvic test.

Side effects might incorporate weighty and delayed periods, draining among periods and pelvic torment.

- Kinds Of Fibroids:

Subserosal fibroids: These are the most widely recognized fibroids. They can drive beyond the uterus into the pelvis. Subserosal fibroids can develop enormously on occasion and in some cases have a tail that connects to the uterus pedunculated fibroid.

Intramural fibroids: These fibroids foster in the strong mass of the uterus.

Submucosal fibroids: These fibroids are extraordinary. They can develop out of the shadows' space inside the uterus and may likewise incorporate a tail.

# Chapter 1

## Who Is At Risk For

## Uterine Fibroids?

Age: Fibroids become more normal as ladies age, particularly during their 30s and 40s and up to menopause. After menopause, fibroids are substantially less liable to frame and generally contract assuming they're available.

Family ancestry: Having a relative with fibroids expands your gamble. On the off chance that a lady's mom had fibroids, her gamble of having them is multiple times higher than normal.

Ethnic beginning: African-American ladies are bound to foster fibroids than different nationalities .

Stoutness: Ladies who are overweight are at higher risk for fibroids. For extremely weighty ladies, the gamble is a few times more prominent than normal.

# Chapter 2

## Symptoms  Of Uterine

## Fibroids?

Most ladies with fibroids will encounter no side effects by any means. In any case, huge or various fibroids can cause the accompanying side effects:

Weighty or drawn out periods
Draining between periods
Pelvic agony and strain
Incessant pee
Low back torment
Torment during intercourse
Trouble getting pregnant

# Chapter 3

## How Are Uterine Fibroids Diagnosed?

Fibroids are most frequently found during an actual test. Your medical care supplier might feel a firm, sporadic (frequently effortless) irregularity during a stomach or pelvic test.

Outputs can affirm a determination. These tests are the two fundamental choices:

- Ultrasound:

Ultrasound is the most usually involved filter for fibroids. It utilizes sound waves to analyze fibroids and includes frequencies (pitch) a lot higher than whatever you can hear. A specialist or expert puts an ultrasound test on the midsection or inside the vagina to assist with checking the uterus and ovaries. It is fast, straightforward and by and large precise. Be that as it may, it depends on the experience and ability of the specialist or expert to deliver great outcomes. Different tests, for example, X-ray might be better for different circumstances, like adenomyosis.

- X-ray:

This imaging test utilizes magnets and radio waves to create pictures. It permits your supplier to acquire a guide of the size, number and area of the fibroids. We can likewise recognize fibroids and adenomyosis, which now and then gets misdiagnosed. We use X-ray to affirm a finding and assist with figuring out which medicines are best for you. X-ray may likewise give a superior choice to related conditions like adenomyosis.

- Hysterosalpingogram (HSG):

Specialists normally utilize a HSG for ladies experiencing difficulty getting pregnant. It actually takes a look at within the uterus (uterine cavity) and fallopian tubes. After a specialist puts a catheter (little cylinder) in the uterus, the specialist gradually infuses a unique color for difference and takes X-beams.

- Hysterosonogram:

Specialists utilize it to see within the uterus. After they place a little catheter inside the uterus, they infuse water while taking a progression of ultrasound pictures. The test can affirm the presence of uterine polyps or intracavitary fibroids that can cause weighty dying.

- Laparoscopy:

For laparoscopy, a specialist makes small entry points in or close to the navel. The specialist then embeds a long, meager instrument (laparoscope) into the mid-region and pelvis. The laparoscope has a splendid light and a camera. It permits your primary care physician to see the uterus and encompassing designs. The view can assist your PCP with deciding whether you have a condition, for example, endometriosis, which can cause pelvic torment.

- Hysteroscopy:

For thought irregularities inside the uterus, a specialist utilizes a long, slender instrument with a camera and light. The specialist goes the instrument through the vagina and cervix into the uterus. No cut is required. The specialist can search for fibroids or endometrial polyps inside the pit of the uterus with this methodology. Your primary care physician may likewise eliminate a few sorts of fibroids during this method.

# Chapter 4

## Will Fibroid Bleeding Stop?

Uterine fibroids could seem like a disturbing condition, however these developments that structure from the muscle tissue of the uterus are quite often non destructive. For some individuals, they cause gentle side effects.

As a matter of fact, it's normal to be asymptomatic and ignorant that you have an uterine fibroid.

All things considered, when side effects do happen, they can go from moderate to serious and include:

Weighty feminine dying

Pelvic agony and strain

Back torment

Pallor

Regular pee in the event that they're coming down on the bladder. Uterine fibroids are most normal in your 30s and 40s however can happen at whatever stage in life. As per the U.S. Office on Ladies' Wellbeing, around 20 to 80 percent Believed wellsprings of ladies foster fibroids by age 50.

A fibroid can be little and particular or develop and duplicate into a few fibroids of changing sizes. In addition, the area isn't the equivalent 100% of the time.

A few fibroids might fill in the uterine wall or be connected to it by a stem-like construction.

Contingent upon the size and area of your fibroids, a specialist might have the option to feel a fibroid during an ordinary pelvic test.

Any other way, they might conclude to do additional testing assuming that you're encountering weighty dying, agony, and changes in feminine cycle, particularly assuming these side effects impede your day to day daily practice or expansion in seriousness or recurrence.

Fibroids will quite often disappear all alone, however at times, as with weighty or agonizing feminine periods, you might require treatment to stop the dying.

# Chapter 5

## Will Fibroid Affect Pregnancy?

Few pregnant ladies have uterine fibroids. Assuming that you are pregnant and have fibroids, they probably won't bring on some issues for you or your child.

During pregnancy, fibroids might increase in size. The vast majority of this development happens from blood streaming to the uterus. Joined with the additional requests put on the body by pregnancy, the development of fibroids might cause distress, sensations of strain, or torment. Fibroids can build the gamble of:

unnatural birth cycle (in which the pregnancy closes before 20 weeks)preterm birth.

Breech birth (in which the child is brought into the world in a position other than head down)

Fibroids don't necessarily fill in pregnancy. In many examinations, most fibroids continued as before. Unconstrained contracting was viewed as in almost 80% of ladies in no less than a half year of pregnancy. Post Pregnancy, redesigning of the uterus might influence fibroids, making a characteristic treatment during the contraceptive years. This might make sense of the defensive impact of equality or number of pregnancies on fibroid risk.

Once in a long while, a huge fibroid can hinder the kickoff of the uterus or hold the child back from passing into the birth waterway. For this situation, the child is conveyed by cesarean birth. Much of the time, even an enormous fibroid will move out of the embryo's way as the uterus extends during pregnancy. Ladies with huge fibroids might have more blood misfortune after conveyance.

Frequently, fibroids needn't bother with being treated during pregnancy. In the event that you are having side effects, for example, torment or uneasiness, your PCP might endorse rest. Once in a while a pregnant lady with fibroids should remain in the emergency clinic for a period due to agony, dying, or compromised preterm work.

Once in a while, a myomectomy might be performed on a pregnant lady. Cesarean birth might be required after myomectomy. Fibroids decline in size after pregnancy much of the time.

A preliminary work isn't suggested in patients at high gamble of uterine burst, incorporating those with past old style or T-formed uterine entry points or broad transfundal uterine medical procedure. Since myomectomy likewise can create a transmural entry point in the uterus, it frequently has been treated in a closely resembling way. There are no clinical preliminaries that explicitly address this issue; in any case, one review reports no uterine cracks in 212 conveyances (83% vaginal) after myomectomy (74).

Pooled information from a few case series of laparoscopic myomectomy including in excess of 750 pregnancies recognized one instance of uterine crack (39, 40, 75-77). Other case reports have depicted the event of uterine break previously and during work (78-80), including interesting case reports of uterine crack remote from term after conventional stomach myomectomy (81, 82). Most obstetricians permit ladies who went through hysteroscopic myomectomy for type O or type I leiomyomas to go through work and conceive an offspring vaginally; nonetheless, there are case reports of uterine break in ladies who experienced uterine hole during hysteroscopy (83-85). Apparently the gamble of uterine burst in pregnancy after laparoscopic or hysteroscopic myomectomy is low. Notwithstanding, in view of the serious idea of this difficulty, a high file of doubt should be kept up with while overseeing pregnancies after this method.

# Chapter 6

## Can Fibroid Shrink

## Without Treatment?

In the event that you've been determined to have uterine fibroids, you've likely pondered, "Might fibroids at any point contract all alone?" Indeed, it relies upon your age and potentially a couple of different elements.

Uterine fibroids appear to fill because of a lady's estrogen creation. What's more, in light of the fact that most fibroids quit developing or may try a psychologist as a lady approaches menopause, your primary care physician might suggest "vigilant pausing," contingent upon your side effects and that you are so near the period of menopause. Vigilant holding up implies that the specialist will screen your side effects to guarantee that there is no sign the fibroids are developing or that your fibroids are bringing about any critical side effects.

Except if fibroids are causing inconvenience, over the top dying, or bladder issues, treatment may not be vital. You ought to be assessed consistently to talk about your side effects and to screen the size of your fibroid and uterus. Your PCP will direct pelvic and stomach assessments to assess size.

Fibroids can increment in size at various rates in every individual. Certain individuals experience quickly developing fibroids with demolishing side effects, while different ladies scarcely notice their fibroids and they progressively vanish all alone. A fibroid-accommodating eating regimen wealthy in natural products, verdant green vegetables, entire milk, and eggs, and low in fats and red meat, may slow the development of fibroids or diminish side effects.

Your general wellbeing and clinical history

The degree of your fibroids

Assumptions for the course of your condition

Your longing to become pregnant

Your capacity to bear explicit meds, methodology, or treatments

Your inclination

There are a few choices for contracting fibroids without medical procedure:

Meds may briefly further develop side effects like torment and draining yet don't cause the fibroids to vanish forever. On the off chance that you have weighty dying, it very well might be useful to investigate drug choices prior to having a strategy (ii). Prescriptions include: (iii)

Nonsteroidal calming drugs, like headache medicine, ibuprofen and naproxen

Hormonal contraceptives, including anti-conception medication pills, vaginal ring, or shots

Tranexamic corrosive, a non hormonal medicine taken during the feminine

cycle

Leuprolide acetic acid derivation, which decreases estrogen creation, making a transitory menopause

Contraceptives might be more proper for more youthful, physically dynamic ladies, though more established ladies might favor nonhormonal treatment (iii). Specialists commonly deter chemical treatment for those with a background marked by cardiovascular failure, stroke, blood clusters, or bosom disease, or smokers age at least 35 (iii). Fortunately, symptoms of these cures are commonly gentle, however a few ladies notice bosom delicacy, weight gain, mind-set changes, or stomach hurts (iii).

Uterine fibroid embolization (UFE) is a negligibly obtrusive treatment choice that has a 85 percent achievement rate (iii). Fitting for ladies who have a developed uterus, the method utilizes imaging to distinguish the course that supplies blood to the fibroids in the uterus. When found, bloodstream to the fibroids is hindered, denying them of supplements and contracting fibroids without medical procedure.

UFE is suggested for ladies who are at present not pregnant and have indicative uterine fibroids like extreme dying, squeezing, pelvic agony, swelling or continuous pee.

Another choice is endometrial removal, which obliterates the covering of the uterus. A possibility for ladies with a typical estimated uterus and little fibroids, removal is suggested for ladies ages 45 and more established on the grounds that pregnancy is as of now not conceivable after this method and can build the gamble of hysterectomy for more youthful ladies (iii). Truth be told, an investigation discovered that roughly 40% of ladies who had endometrial removal later had a hysterectomy (iii).

# Chapter 7

## Can Fibroid Cause

## Miscarriage?

Most ladies experience no side effects of fibroids, however they can create huge issues in uncommon cases.

The probability of confusions happening relies upon elements like the position.

Assuming that fibroids are available during pregnancy, it can in some cases lead to issues with the advancement of the child or troubles during work.
Ladies with fibroids might encounter stomach (stomach) torment during pregnancy, and there's a gamble of untimely work.

In the event that enormous fibroids block the vagina, a cesarean segment (where the child is conveyed through a cut in the stomach and belly) might be vital.
In uncommon cases, fibroids can cause an unnatural birth cycle (the deficiency of pregnancy during the initial 23 weeks).

Your GP or birthing specialist will actually want to offer you additional data and guidance in the event that you have fibroids and are pregnant.

Fruitlessness
Fruitlessness (the failure to become pregnant) may happen in situations where a lady has huge fibroids.

Fibroids can at times forestall a prepared egg connecting itself to the covering of the belly, or forestall sperm arriving at the egg, yet this is intriguing.
Assuming you have a submucosal fibroid (a fibroid that develops from the muscle wall into the depression of your belly), it might hinder a fallopian tube, making it harder for you to become pregnant. The fallopian tubes interface the ovaries (where the egg is delivered) to the belly.

# Chapter 8

## Can Fibroid Shrink After Menopause?

Fibroids need the chemical estrogen to develop. After menopause, estrogen levels decline decisively, which for the most part decreases the gamble of creating fibroids.

Much of the time, fibroids psychologists cause less side effects after menopause.

Be that as it may, certain individuals may not see a lessening in side effects.

Chemical treatment (HT) intends to keep up with levels of estrogen and progesterone during perimenopause and after menopause. Hence, fibroids might keep on developing.

A few medicines for fibroids mean an individual can presently not become pregnant. Frequently, this isn't an issue after menopause. Nonetheless, it could be a considerationTrusted Hotspot for any individual who has passed menopause and is thinking about pregnancy through helped regenerative innovations.

- Side effects

As indicated by the Workplace on Ladies' HealthTrusted Source, fibroids can fluctuate from the size of an apple seed to that of a grapefruit. An individual can have one or many. Consequently, certain individuals have no side effects, while others can encounter serious distress.

The side effects of fibroids frequently continue as before no matter what an individual's age.

- They can include:

Weighty draining during the regenerative years and draining that can continueTrusted Source after menopause

Extended mid-region

A sensations of completion in the lower mid-region

Torment during sex

Tension on the bladder or insides
Incessant pee
Lower back torment.

Fibroids are harmless by definition, yet in uncommon cases, a development that gives off an impression of being a fibroid contains destructive cells. This occurs in less than 1 in 1,000Trusted Source fibroids. Besides, the aggravation and inconvenience of fibroids can seriously influence an individual's general prosperity and personal satisfaction, including their capacity to work or perform routine exercises.
Hence, an individual ought to look for clinical guidance on the off chance that they have any side effects of fibroids.

- Treatment

Medicines for fibroids can go from a "watch and pause" approach on the off chance that there are no side effects to a myomectomy in the event that side effects are serious.

- Factors a specialist will consider while settling on a treatment plan include:

Size of the fibroids
Area of the fibroids
An individual's age
The presence and seriousness of side effects
Before menopause, fibroids can influence fruitfulness. After menopause, the vast majority don't require treatment for fibroids except if the fibroids are enormous or they have serious side effects. Here are some optionsTrusted Source a specialist might suggest.

- Watch and pause

Many individuals decide not to have treatment for their fibroids since they will more often than not shrivel or disappear after menopause. Notwithstanding, it is as yet vital to check in with a specialist routinely to check in the event that they have developed.

- Medicine

Assuming the fibroids are causing side effects, specialists might suggest drugs.

Nonsteroidal mitigating drugs (NSAIDs), like ibuprofen or acetaminophen, may assist with easing torment.

Gonadotropin-delivering chemical agonists (GnRHa), like Lupron, can assist with contracting fibroids and make them simpler to eliminate during a medical procedure. An individual can take GnRHa drugs by infusion, nasal splash, or as an embed.

Different choices includeTrusted Source oral conception prevention pills or having an intrauterine gadget (IUD).
- Medical procedure

Medical procedure might be a choice assuming fibroids are enormous, or side effects are extreme.
- Myomectomy:This method eliminates fibroids however leaves the sound tissue of the uterus. New fibroids can be created after a myomectomy. Pregnancy might in any case be conceivable after this medical procedure.

Medical procedures can be open or hysteroscopic, contingent upon the degree of the fibroids. In a hysteroscopy, a specialist insertsTrusted Source along, a flimsy gadget through the vagina and cervix into the uterus. A camera on the finish of the gadget empowers the specialist to see within the uterus. During this strategy, the specialist can utilize a similar instrument to eliminate fibroids.
Hysterectomy:A hysterectomy is a methodology to eliminate the uterus. On the off chance that medical procedure occurs around menopause, the specialist may likewise eliminate the ovaries.
A hysterectomy will end the side effects of uterine fibroids, making it a reasonable decision for somebody with serious side effects who doesn't want to have kids.
Specialists play out a hysterectomy utilizing open or laparoscopic medical procedure. They may likewise involve a vaginal methodology in a technique known as a laparoscopic-helped vaginal hysterectomy.

Contingent upon the sort of a medical procedure, recuperation can take up to 6 weeksTrusted Source.

In the US, fibroids are the most widely recognized justification for a hysterectomy, representing 37% of hysterectomies every year.

- Endometrial ablation:In endometrial removal, a specialist eliminates or obliterates the covering of the uterus. This can assist with overseeing side effects.

It is feasible to become pregnant after this technique, yet specialists don't inform them because of the gamble with respect to pregnancy misfortune and different issues. Individuals ought to possibly go through removal assuming that they are done intending to have kids.

- Myolysis:In myolysis, a specialist insertsTrusted Source a needle into a fibroid and passes either an electric flow or freezing system through the needle to obliterate the fibroid tissue. It is likewise known asTrusted Source radiofrequency removal.

Uterine fibroid or vein embolization

Uterine fibroid embolization additionally called uterine corridor embolization includes obstructing the veins that carry blood to the fibroid. The fibroid ought to recoil, however pregnancy may not be prudent confided in source form .

# Chapter 9

## Will Fibroid Pain Go Away?

For certain ladies, the aggravation from fibroids can be serious. Aside from weighty feminine draining and delayed periods, fibroids can cause:

Dull, constant pelvic tension and agony
lower back torment
stomach expanding and bulging
torment with periods or sex
They might cause you to feel like you really want to regularly pee. The aggravation might travel every which way or happen just during sex or monthly cycle. It could be sharp or a dull hurt. Side effects can likewise change contingent upon the area, size, and number of fibroids you have.

- The side effects of fibroids might be like other pelvic issues, for example,

Endometriosis
Adenomyosis
Pelvic disease
On the off chance that you have pelvic torment that won't disappear, weighty and extensive stretches, and issues with peeing, seeing a specialist for a right diagnosis is significant.
The aggravation and tension side effects related with uterine fibroids for the most part result from the heaviness of the actual fibroid squeezing or laying on the pelvic organs, as opposed to the actual fibroid harming. Ultrasound tests are useful to assess the size and area of a fibroid. They can assist your primary care physician with knowing whether the fibroid is answerable for the aggravation you might have.

You might have the option to oversee side effects with non-prescription drugs and home cures. This is particularly obvious in the event that you just have minor side effects that aren't influencing your everyday life.

- Home cures include:

Nonsteroidal calming drugs, like ibuprofen, particularly during your period
warming cushions or warm packs
rub
There are likewise a few home cures that might assist with lessening different side effects of fibroids:

Eat a solid eating regimen wealthy in natural products, vegetables, entire grains, and lean meats, and keep away from red meat, refined starches and sweet food varieties as these may demolish fibroids
polish off dairy items, like milk, yogurt, and cheddar, no less than one time each day
limit liquor
take nutrient and mineral enhancements, including iron and B nutrients, to assist with forestalling weakness brought about by weighty dying
work-out routinely and keep a sound weight.

# Chapter 10

## What do fibroids look like?

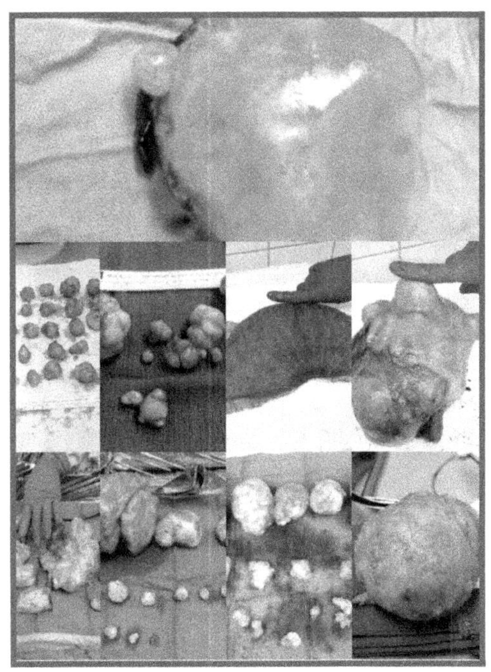

# Chapter 11

## Why Do Fibroids Causes

## Heavy Bleeding?

Could it be said that you are encountering weighty draining or pelvic agony? The reason could be uterine fibroids. These non-malignant growths can prompt weighty draining during your period or spotting between cycles. It's critical to perceive the indications of uterine fibroids, as well as realize that there are treatment choices that will assist you with returning to the individual you were before your fibroids. Fibroids, otherwise called uterine leiomyomas, are harmless developments that create inside or on the walls of the uterus. With regards to weighty dying, fibroids can assume a huge part. The development of fibroids can prompt an augmentation of the uterus, which upsets the ordinary equilibrium of hormonal guidelines during the period. This disturbance can bring about an expansion in the creation of specific chemicals, for example, estrogen, which can invigorate the development of the endometrium (the coating of the uterus). Accordingly, the endometrium becomes thicker and greater than expected, prompting heavier and delayed feminine dying. Furthermore, fibroids can cause switches in the veins up the uterus, making them more vulnerable to dying. The mix of these elements adds to the appearance of weighty draining in ladies with fibroids, frequently bringing about critical uneasiness and disturbance to their regular routines.

- Fibroids and Sporadic Dying

For ladies who truly do encounter uterine fibroid side effects, the most well-known is unpredictable or weighty dying. Strange draining is anything beyond your period, on the off chance that your stream is fundamentally heavier than typical, or on the other hand assuming you experience any repetition during menopause. This kind of draining without anyone else doesn't necessarily in every case show a difficult condition, however it's frequently connected to uterine fibroids.

On the off chance that you have uterine fibroids, you might see these side effects:

Weighty, delayed periods enduring 10+ days
Sporadic dying
Pelvic strain or torment
Regular pee or trouble purging the bladder
Blockage or other digestive issues
Back or leg torment
Trouble getting pregnant
Swelling or jutting paunch

A large number of our patients have let us know that weighty, capricious draining was the game changer in deciding to look for fibroid treatment. Because of the way that each circumstance is unique, a few ladies may not encounter weighty, delayed dying. Assuming you have seen that you are utilizing more ladylike cleanliness items than ordinary, it could be a sign of uterine fibroids. Periods enduring longer than 10 days out of each month, or reliably draining between feminine cycles, isn't typical.

Ladies with fibroids who are going through menopause frequently see an improvement in unusual dying. This is on the grounds that fibroids shrivel when estrogen levels drop during menopause. Nonetheless, few postmenopausal ladies will in any case encounter weighty draining from uterine fibroids and search for a treatment cholce.

• Weighty draining because of Fibroids and Weakness
The weighty draining brought about by fibroids can prompt a condition known as sickliness. Pallor happens when there is a diminishing in the quantity of red platelets or a low degree of hemoglobin in the blood. Hemoglobin is answerable for conveying oxygen to different pieces of the body. Over the top and delayed feminine draining related with fibroids can bring about a critical loss

of blood, prompting a diminishing in red platelets and hemoglobin levels. This can eventually bring about sickliness, prompting side effects like exhaustion, shortcoming, windedness, wooziness, and fair skin. Weakness can fundamentally influence an individual's personal satisfaction, making it vital to address the hidden reason for weighty dying, like fibroids, to really forestall or oversee paleness. Legitimate finding, treatment, and the board of fibroids can assist with easing weighty dying, lessen the gamble of sickliness, and reestablish generally wellbeing and prosperity.

- Treatment for Fibroids and Strange Dying

In the event that you have fibroids and unpredictable dying, you're in good company. Different ladies have strolled a similar way, and there's a treatment choice that can assist you with feeling such as yourself once more. We comprehend how disappointing and distressing flighty, weighty draining can be. USA Fibroid Focuses offers Uterine Fibroid Embolization (UFE), a treatment that can assist with easing your weighty draining and other uterine fibroid side effects. UFE is a short term method that mainly requires around 30-45 minutes.

# Chapter 12

## What Causes Fibroid?

Specialists don't have the foggiest idea about the reason for uterine fibroids, however research and clinical experience highlight these elements:

Hereditary changes. Numerous fibroids contain changes in quantities that vary from those in regular uterine muscle cells.

Chemicals. Estrogen and progesterone, two chemicals that animate improvement of the uterine covering during each monthly cycle in anticipation of pregnancy, seem to advance the development of fibroids.

Fibroids contain more estrogen and progesterone receptors than normal uterine muscle cells do. Fibroids will more often than not contract after menopause because of a reduction in chemical creation.

Other development factors. Substances that assist the body with keeping up with tissues, for example, insulin-like development factor, may influence fibroid development.

- Extracellular network (ECM). ECM is the material that makes cells remain together, similar to mortar between blocks. ECM is expanded in fibroids and makes them sinewy. ECM likewise stores development factors and causes biologic changes in the actual cells.

Specialists accept that uterine fibroids create from an immature microorganism in the smooth solid tissue of the uterus (myometrium). A solitary cell partitions over and over, in the long run making a firm, rubbery mass unmistakable from neighboring tissue.

The development examples of uterine fibroids differ: they might develop gradually or quickly, or they might continue as before size. A few fibroids go through development sprays, and some might shrivel all alone.

Numerous fibroids that have been available during pregnancy shrivel or vanish after pregnancy, as the uterus returns to its standard size.

- Risk factors

There are not many realized risk factors for uterine fibroids, other than being a lady of regenerative age. Factors that can affect fibroid improvement include:

- Race.

Although all ladies of contraceptive age could foster fibroids, people of color are bound to have fibroids than are ladies of other racial gatherings. Likewise, people of color have fibroids at more youthful ages, and they're additionally prone to have more or bigger fibroids, alongside more-extreme side effects.

Heredity. On the off chance that your mom or sister had fibroids, you're at an expanded hazard of creating them.

- Different elements.

Beginning your period at an early age; weight; a lack of vitamin D; having an eating routine higher in red meat and lower in green vegetables, foods grown from the ground; and drinking liquor, including brew, seem to expand your gamble of creating fibroids.

- Confusions

Although uterine fibroids normally aren't perilous, they can cause uneasiness and may prompt complexities like a drop in red platelets (iron deficiency), which causes exhaustion, from weighty blood misfortune. Once in a while, a bonding is required because of blood misfortune.

- Pregnancy and fibroids

Fibroids typically don't obstruct getting pregnant. In any case, it's conceivable that fibroids, particularly submucosal fibroids, could cause fruitlessness or pregnancy misfortune.

Fibroids may likewise raise the gamble of specific pregnancy confusions, like placental suddenness, fetal development limitation and preterm conveyance.

- Counteraction

Despite the fact that analysts keep on concentrating on the reasons for fibroid cancers, minimal logical proof is accessible on the best way to forestall them. Forestalling uterine fibroids may not be imaginable, yet just a little level of these growths require treatment. However, by pursuing sound way of life decisions, for example, keeping a solid weight and eating foods grown from the ground, you might have the option to diminish your fibroid risk.

Likewise, some examination recommends that utilizing hormonal contraceptives might be related with a lower hazard of fibroids.

# Chapter 13

## How Fibroid Surgery

## Is Done

Uterine fibroids are developments in your uterus. Since they're commonly not harmful, you can conclude whether you need to have them eliminated.

You may not require a medical procedure on the off chance that your fibroids don't irritate you. Nonetheless, you should seriously mull over a medical procedure in the event that your fibroids cause:

Weighty feminine dying
Draining between periods
Torment or tension in your lower stomach
incessant pee
Inconvenience discharging your bladder
Medical procedure could likewise be a choice if you have any desire to get pregnant later on. Here and there fibroids can build your gamble of having a premature delivery or inconveniences during your pregnancy.

In the event that you choose to have fibroid medical procedure, you have two choices:

Myomectomy
Hysterectomy
Medical procedure can ease your fibroid side effects, however it accompanies gambles. Your PCP will talk you through your choices. Together, you can choose whether to have a technique and, provided that this is true, which one to have.

Sorts of fibroid medical procedure
There are two sorts of fibroid systems. Which one you have relies upon:

The size of your fibroids
The quantity of fibroids you have
where in your uterus they're found
whether you need to have kids.
Myomectomy
Myomectomy eliminates your fibroids and can ease draining and different side effects. This medical procedure is a choice assuming you might want to have kids from now on, or on the other hand if you need to save your uterus for another explanation.

Around 80 to 90 percent of ladies who have a myomectomy get help from their side effects or see their side effects decreased. The fibroids will not recover after a medical procedure, yet you might foster new fibroids. Up to 33 percent of ladies who have this medical procedure will require a recurrent method in no less than 5 years since they develop new fibroids.

This medical procedure should be possible in one of three ways, contingent upon the number, size, and area of your fibroids. You'll be under broad sedation for these systems.
- Hysteroscopy

This strategy is more powerful for ladies with more modest and less fibroids. Hysteroscopy can likewise eliminate fibroids that have developed within your uterus.
During the method, the specialist embeds a long, slight, lit telescope through your vagina and cervix into your uterus. Liquid is infused into your uterus to extend it and assist your primary care physician with seeing your fibroids.
Then, at that point, the specialist utilizes a gadget to cut or obliterate your fibrolds. The fibroid pieces wash out with the liquid that was utilized to fill your uterus.
With hysteroscopy you might return home that very day as your medical procedure.
- Stomach myomectomy

This technique, otherwise called a laparotomy, is better for enormous fibroids, yet it leaves a greater scar than the other two sorts of myomectomy. For this method, your specialist makes a cut in your lower midsection and eliminates your fibroids.

After stomach myomectomy, you'll remain in the medical clinic for one to three days. Complete recuperation requires 2 to about a month and a half.

- Laparoscopy

Laparoscopy is utilized for ladies who have more modest and less fibroids. During laparoscopy, your specialist makes two little cuts in your midsection. A telescope is embedded into one of the openings to assist your primary care physician with seeing inside your pelvis and around your uterus. An instrument is embedded into the other opening to eliminate your fibroids.

Your specialist might cut your fibroids into little pieces prior to eliminating them. In automated laparoscopy, your specialist utilizes mechanical arms to carry out the technique

Laparoscopic methods might require a short-term emergency clinic stay however have a quicker recuperation than stomach myomectomy.

- Hysterectomy

Hysterectomy eliminates part or the entirety of your uterus. This methodology might be a choice in the event that you have a ton of fibroids, they're enormous, and you're not wanting to have kids.

The specialist can eliminate your uterus in maybe a couple ways: Laparotomy or stomach hysterectomy. Your specialist makes a cut in the lower mid-region and eliminates your uterus.

- Vaginal hysterectomy. The specialist eliminates your uterus through your vagina. This approach may not work for exceptionally enormous fibroids.

- Laparoscopic hysterectomy. The specialist embeds the instruments and eliminates the uterus through little entry points. This method should be possible mechanically.

The specialist might leave your ovaries and cervix set up. Then, at that point, you will keep on creating female chemicals.

Complete recuperation from a stomach hysterectomy requires 6 to about two months. Recuperation from laparoscopic and vaginal hysterectomy is speedier.

Hysterectomy is the main medical procedure that fixes uterine fibroids and completely eases their side effects. In any case, you can never again have kids.

- Endometrial removal

Endometrial removal isn't a medical procedure, however this strategy is still negligibly obtrusive. It annihilates the covering of your uterus. It works best in ladies who have little fibroids found near the uterus. Removal doesn't eliminate your fibroids, yet it eases weighty dying. It's additionally not for ladies who need to get pregnant later on. Endometrial removal should be possible in your primary care physician's office or an emergency clinic. Now and again it's performed simultaneously using a different methodology.

You might get general sedation during the system. Or on the other hand, you might get spinal or epidural sedation to numb you starting from the waist.

During the strategy, the specialist will embed an extraordinary instrument into your uterus and consume off your uterine coating utilizing one of these techniques:

- An electric flow

an inflatable loaded up with warmed liquid

high-energy radio waves (radio recurrence)

a virus test

microwave energy

warmed liquid

You can return home around the same time as your strategy. Your recuperation time will rely upon the kind of removal you had. Endometrial removal is effectiveTrusted Hotspot for easing weighty draining from fibroids.

Medical procedure and ripeness

What fibroid medical procedure means for your ripeness relies upon which sort of system you have. You can not convey a kid after hysterectomy since your uterus will be taken out. You ought to have the option to consider after myomectomy.

After a removal, you probably will not have the option to get pregnant, yet you ought to utilize contraceptionTrusted Source following the method. This is on the grounds that the technique eliminates the endometrial covering where the egg would ordinarily embed. On the off chance that you do imagine, you'll be at higher gamble of having an unsuccessful labor too other serious pregnancy difficulties.

Assuming that you have a methodology that permits you to get pregnant later on, you might have to stand by 90 days or more prior to attempting to imagine to be certain your uterus has completely mended.

- Other treatment choices

Medical procedure isn't the best way to treat fibroids. Certain meds can be utilized to assist with diminishing the side effects that accompany fibroids, yet these choices won't dispose of your fibroids. Different choices include:

- Drugs

Nonsteroidal calming drugs like ibuprofen (Advil, Motrin) and naproxen (Aleve, Naprosyn) can assist with easing torment.

Anti-conception medication pills and different sorts of hormonal contraception strategies, for example, progestin-delivering IUDs can assist with weighty dying.

Against hormonal medications like progestin or danazol block estrogen to treat fibroids.

Gonadotropin-delivering chemical agonists (Lupron, Synarel) block the creation of estrogen and progesterone, and put you into impermanent menopause, which recoils your fibroids. Your PCP could endorse these to make your fibroids more modest before medical procedure.

- Tranexamic corrosive (Lysteda) decreases weighty draining during your periods.

Harmless strategies

X-ray directed centered ultrasound medical procedure utilizes sound waves directed by a X-ray scanner to warm and obliterate your fibroids through your skin.

Uterine course embolization infuses small particles into the corridors that supply your uterus. Removing blood stream to the fibroids makes them shrivel.

Myolysis, for example, the Acessa methodology, utilizes an electric flow or intensity to obliterate your fibroids and the veins that supply them.

Cryomyolysis is like myolysis, then again, actually it freezes the fibroids.

- Chances

These strategies are protected, however they can have gambles, for example,

dying

disease

the requirement for a recurrent system

harm to organs in your mid-region, like your bladder or gut

scar tissue in your midsection, which can shape groups that tight spot organs and tissue together

entrail or urinary issues

richness issues

pregnancy complexities

intriguing opportunity that you'll require a hysterectomy

Laparoscopy causes less draining and different complexities than laparotomy.

- Benefits

Fibroid medical procedure and endometrial removal can assist with alleviating side effects like weighty draining and stomach torment. Eliminating your uterus gives a super durable answer for most fibroid-related side effects.

# Chapter 14

## Where Do Fibroids Grow?

Submucosal fibroids develop inside the uterine pit. Here a developing child lives. Fibroids here can cause extremely weighty feminine dying, fruitfulness issues, and issues with conveying or conveying a youngster. Huge fibroids in this space can likewise broaden the uterus to look like outrageous weight gain or a pregnancy-type stomach.

Intramural fibroids develop inside the solid mass of the uterus. This is the solid region that agrees while conceiving an offspring. Fibroids filling in this space can cause pelvic torment, strange feminine cycles, and awkward strain. An uterine wall loaded with fibroids frequently implies serious and continuous squeezing.

Subserosal fibroids develop outward mass of the uterus. This produces fibroid side effects like back agony and bladder tension as developing fibroids press on sensitive spots or potentially different organs in the body.

Pedunculated fibroids portray fibroids that develop on stalks, similar to mushrooms. They can rise up out of either within or outside uterine walls. A contorted or blocked tail will cause serious pelvic torment.

For what reason are Fibroids Filling in my Uterus?
Albeit certain variables are related with fibroid improvement, there is no plainly characterized because'. The condition is very normal. 1-4 ladies over age 40 have fibroids. However, fibroids are additionally tracked down in more youthful ladies (as a rule during pregnancy). And that's only the tip of the iceberg and more ladies in their 30's, who aren't pregnant and don't fit an exemplary 'fibroid-inclined' profile, appear to be encountering the condition.

So what's really happening here? Clinical examinations have previously connected fibroid improvement to a flood in estrogen levels. Estrogen spikes, like in pregnancy or perimenopause, will more often than not be high-fibroid times. Be that as it may, fibroids are likewise happening in young ladies who aren't pregnant. In postmenopausal ladies, where estrogen levels ought to be genuinely low. What's more, in mid-30's ladies, who customarily aren't considered in danger for this condition.

# Chapter 15

## Common Risk Factors

## for Fibroids

Heredity. Know whether your mom had fibroids or grandma had fibroids. Do your aunties, sisters or other female family members have fibroids? There's an excellent opportunity you will as well. There hasn't been a quality disconnected or connected with fibroid improvement. Furthermore, not much data with regards to following investigations. In any case, clinical proof noted by OB/GYNs regarding this matter proposes that fibroids run in families.

- Identity.

African American ladies are the ethnic gathering probably going to have fibroids. Ladies of Asian plummet are the most improbable. Nobody knows why. While fibroids show up in ladies, all things considered, measurable proof focuses on identity as a force to be reckoned with.

- Diet.

You've most likely heard that dispensing with red meat makes a difference. Likewise soy-based items. Additionally certain estrogen-rich food varieties, similar to sweet potatoes. Chemicals that happen normally (and not so normally) are ample in our food supply. While no substantial connection has been laid out, there is motivation to accept diet might add to the presence of fibroids.

- Weight-gain.

It's obviously true that fat cells in the body discharge substances that impersonate estrogen. Being overweight could make sense why more youthful ladies, who aren't normally aren't considered in danger of fibroids, actually foster them. What's more, why post-menopausal ladies, whose chemical levels ought to be low, are confronting fibroid issues.

# Chapter 16

## Where Is Fibroid Location

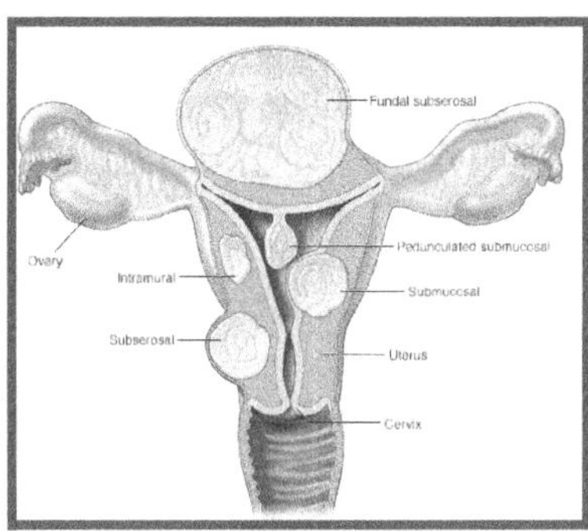

# Chapter 17

## Do Fibroids Causes Pain

## In Specific Areas?

Uterine fibroids can cause torment and uneasiness in regions all through a lady's body. An exploration investigation discovered that ladies with fibroids were bound to report moderate or serious torment during sex, and, surprisingly, noncyclic pelvic torment (pelvic agony unassociated with different circumstances) than ladies without fibroids.

The seriousness of side effects relies upon the size, area, and number of fibroids present. The following are a portion of the normal reasons for torment from various sorts of uterine fibroids:

Intramural and submucosal fibroids inside your uterus can twist its shape

Subserosal fibroids situated outwardly of your uterus can press against your bladder, rectum, or spinal nerves, causing back torment, stomach strain, and enlarging

Pedunculated fibroids are joined by tail like developments either inside or beyond your uterus that might become bent

Fibroids can come down on the sciatic nerve causing back torment which can likewise transmit through the posterior, hips, and legs, as well as agony in uterus and lower back

Assuming you are encountering agony or inconvenience because of fibroids, it could be an ideal opportunity to investigate your treatment choices for how to dispose of fibroid back torment. Assuming you are pondering, "Where is fibroid torment felt?" consider the accompanying fibroid torment areas.

- Stomach Agony

Ladies with huge fibroids frequently experience pelvic and additional stomach inconvenience. This might present as extreme torment limited to a particular spot or can be gentle yet influence a bigger region of the body.

Fibroids can likewise cause stomach or gut torment that adversely influences your stomach related framework. On the off chance that a fibroid is sufficiently huge, it can push down on the rectum, making solid discharges troublesome which might cause blockage. Unnecessary rectal strain because of clogging can likewise bring about hemorrhoids, which happen because of enlarged veins in the butt.

Fibroids can expand the aggravation from feminine squeezing, making it more extreme than typical. This aggravation may likewise endure longer than expected as fibroids can broaden your period. As the fibroid develops, it can enlarge your uterus, making your midsection seem bigger than ordinary.

- Back Agony

One of the areas where fibroid torment is believed is toward the back. Fibroids can press against the nerves in the lower back or push on the muscles, which might bring about torment. Bigger fibroids as a rule are the guilty party as little fibroids are less inclined to have sufficient strain to bring about torment outside the uterus.

- Leg Agony

Fibroids can cause leg torment assuming they press on nerves or muscles. This typically occurs with bigger fibroids and those that develop outwardly of the uterus. Torment in the lower back can transmit down the leg, causing far and wide uneasiness.

- Head

Ladies with fibroids experience cerebral pains because of paleness. Lack of iron weakness, a typical side effect of fibroids, is a condition wherein you need sufficient red platelets to convey satisfactory oxygen all through your body.

In the event that you experience back, leg, or pelvic agony, we prescribe talking with a fibroid expert to decide its fundamental reason. The solution to the inquiry, "Do fibroids cause torment?" is "yes." However you can seek help with fibroid treatment.

# Chapter 18

## Why Fibroid Pain

## During Pregnancy?

Most ladies who have been determined to have fibroids proceed to have typical pregnancies, however here and there they can cause difficulties.

Issues During the Principal Trimester
Most fibroids don't develop while you're pregnant, however assuming it happens it doubtlessly will be during your initial 3 months (first trimester). That is on the grounds that fibroids need a chemical called estrogen to develop. Your body delivers a greater amount of it when you're pregnant.
The essential issues that could happen are:

Draining and torment. In an investigation of in excess of 4,500 ladies, scientists viewed that as 11% of the ones who had fibroids likewise had died, and 59% had simply torment. Yet, 30% of the ladies had both draining and torment during their most memorable trimester. Unnatural birth cycle. Ladies with fibroids are considerably more prone to lose during early pregnancy than ladies without them (14% versus 7.6%). Furthermore, assuming you have different or extremely huge fibroids, your possibilities go up significantly more.

Second and Third Trimesters
As your uterus extends to account for your child, it can push against your fibroids. This can cause various issues during your pregnancy:
- Torment:

This is the most well-known side effect of fibroids, particularly on the off chance that they're enormous. Some of the time, fibroids curve, which can cause squeezing and inconvenience. Different times, the

fibroid grows out of its blood supply, becomes red and bites the dust. This cycle, called "red degeneration," can cause extreme stomach torments. At times, it can prompt premature delivery.
Over-the-counter prescriptions like acetaminophen (Tylenol) can facilitate your aggravation. Yet, keep away from non-steroidal mitigating drugs (NSAIDs) like ibuprofen (Advil) early and later in your pregnancy since it might make you lose, diminish how much amniotic liquid, or cause heart issues in your child.

- Placental suddenness:

Continuous examinations appear to show that pregnant ladies with fibroids have a lot more prominent possibility of placental unexpectedness than ladies without fibroids. That implies your placenta tears from the mass of your uterus before your child is conveyed. It's intense on the grounds that your child will not get sufficient oxygen and you can have weighty dying. You could go into shock.

Preterm conveyance: On the off chance that you have fibroids, you're bound to convey preterm - - meaning your child is brought into the world before 37 weeks of pregnancy than ladies without fibroids.

# Chapter 19

## Can Fibroid Prevent

## Pregnancy?

Around 80% of ladies will have had a fibroid when they turn 50. They're normal developments that foster in the uterus, and they're for the most part effortless. Be that as it may, some of the time fibroids can slow down ripeness and make it more challenging to get pregnant.

At our far reaching OB/GYN facilities in Cranston, Provision, and Smithfield, Rhode Island, A. Michael Coppa, MD and our group are here to assist you with exploring fruitlessness and having a solid pregnancy. Converse with Dr. Coppa about what fibroids could mean for your possibilities of getting pregnant.

Fibroids are normal. More often than not, they don't influence your capacity to get pregnant. Be that as it may, on the off chance that you have a great deal of fibroids or they're submucosal fibroids, they might influence richness.

Also,having fibroids doesn't obstruct ovulation, yet submucosal fibroids can make it harder for your uterus to help origination and keep up with pregnancy. At times, this sort of fibroid can cause barrenness or pregnancy misfortune.

Dr. Coppa determined fibroids to have a pelvic test that could incorporate an ultrasound or X-ray. Contingent upon the size and area of your fibroids, he suggests a treatment plan that is ideal for you. Assuming you're pregnant or attempting to consider, it's vital to intently screen the fibroids.

Having fibroids while pregnant can build your gamble of intricacies during work and conveyance, including the probability that you'll require a cesarean segment. Your gamble of placental suddenness or preterm conveyance could likewise be higher on the off chance that you have fibroids.

# Chapter 20

## Can Fibroids Cause

## Back Pain?

Did you have any idea that occasionally, fibroids cause back torment? Assuming you've been determined to have fibroids, you likely realize that they are non-destructive cancers that fill in your uterus. What's more, chances are, you encountered some fibroid side effects before that conclusion. Perhaps your periods were truly weighty. Or on the other hand maybe you encountered constant pelvic agony.

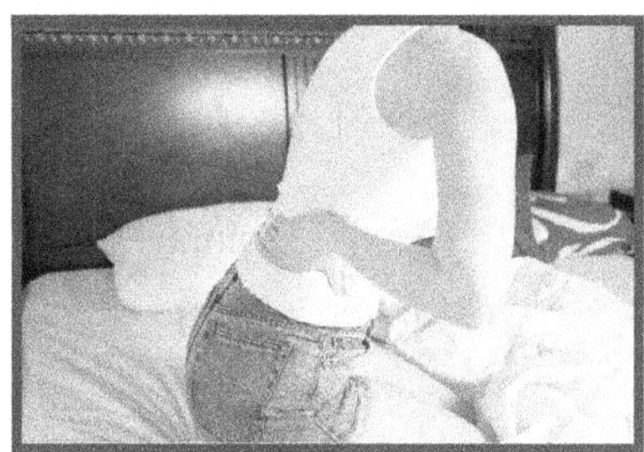

In any case, assuming your fibroid side effects incorporate back, leg and stomach torment, you could ponder: how should uterine developments hurt in such countless different spots?
Just relax, you're in good company. Diffuse torment is a typical fibroid side effect. That is on the grounds that fibroids can come down on your sciatic nerve, leaving you with back torment, as well as emanating torment in your hips, bum, and legs. It tends to be alarming when you feel these side effects everywhere, except we're here to assist you with understanding how uterine fibroids spread

side effects to the remainder of your body. Furthermore, why fibroids
cause back torment.

# Chapter 21

Relief from Fibroid Pain

Without Surgery

At the point when fibroid torment influences so many body parts, it can obstruct your everyday existence. Assuming you're there, you're probably exploring fibroid treatment choices. Also, you genuinely must realize that medical procedure isn't your main choice.

While certain ladies will decide to go through myomectomy (careful evacuation of fibroid cancers), you might wish to keep away from this intrusive strategy. Provided that this is true, ensure you look into uterine fibroid embolization (UFE), an insignificantly intrusive method we perform at our Houston fibroids practice.

It's not unexpected a preferable decision over hysterectomy, which triggers significant incidental effects, including bone misfortune, cognitive decline

With this methodology, our doctors use catheters to get to your fibroid's blood supply, removing the stream with a long-lasting store of embolic material. After UFE, your fibroids therapist or even vanish totally. Also, when that occurs, you will probably encounter help from back and leg torment, alongside other undesirable fibroid side effects.

In any case, that is not all: on the grounds that UFE is negligibly obtrusive, you can keep away from general sedation and probably won't have to remain in the clinic short-term. Furthermore, in light of the fact that UFE just requires a little entry point in your arm, your recuperation time is a lot quicker than with a strategy like hysterectomy or even myomectomy. Furthermore, UFE systems have an exceptionally high achievement rate, meaning your help ought to endure.

# Chapter 22

## Can Fibroid Tumors Be Cancerous?

Uterine fibroids are not malignant growth. They are harmless growths that foster on uterine tissue, and they are extremely normal. In the US, an expected 26 million ladies between the ages of 15 and 50 have uterine fibroids.

Most ladies with fibroids experience no side effects. Yet, for the people who do, stressing whether your uterine fibroids may be harmful is ordinary. All things considered, the side effects of fibroid growths are like some uterine disease side effects.

Fortunately uterine fibroids are seldom destructive. Less than one of every 1,000 fibroids end up harboring malignant growth.

Likewise, uterine fibroids themselves are not harmful.

Nonetheless, harmful development can conceal inside a fibroid. In the event that is the situation, it's basic to seek therapy immediately as this kind of malignant growth can spread rapidly.

Eventually, every lady ought to understand what uterine fibroids are and what to do assuming they're encountering side effects showing any kind of development on the uterus. Grasping uterine fibroids, malignant growth, and the distinctions can engage you to do whatever it may take to safeguard your contraceptive wellbeing.

# Chapter 23

## Can Uterine Fibroids

## Harm My Pregnancy?

Huge uterine fibroids, which should be visible on ultrasounds, may build a few dangers during pregnancy.
From the get-go in pregnancy, it's normal to determine a patient to have previous circumstances that could cause worry during the following nine months.

While diabetes and hypertension are normal worries we analyze during pregnancy, 1% to 10% of hopeful mothers are found to have uterine fibroids - unusual however noncancerous tissue developments inside the uterus - during a pre-birth ultrasound. For some this is another finding, yet numerous ladies are as of now mindful they have them.

Uterine fibroids are normal. By age 35, 40% to 60% of ladies will have fostered these developments, which can cause stomach massiveness and weighty or difficult periods.
All things being equal, the finding can be disturbing for certain patients. I have odd tissue developing close to my child? What's the significance here for my pregnancy?

While there is a lot of exploration on fibroids in nonpregnant patients, information is restricted on what fibroids can mean for pregnancy. Fortunately, we really do realize that most patients with fibroids will have an unremarkable pregnancy and conveyance.
Having a couple of little fibroids is seldom reason to worry. In any case, contingent upon the area of your fibroids, the number of you have, and whether they are huge - fibroids can go from the size of a

coin to a b-ball - we will screen for specific circumstances that can create issues during pregnancy.

- Strange placenta:

Fibroids have been related with placenta previa (implantation of the placenta over the cervix) and placental unexpectedness (untimely partition of the placenta from the uterus). Your primary care physician can utilize ultrasound to actually take a look at the placenta during pregnancy.

- Fibroid development:

Exploration recommends that around 66% of fibroids will develop or recoil during pregnancy. Assuming development happens, it's normally during the principal trimester. Your Ob/Gyn might check the size of your fibroids by means of ultrasound to screen changes and assess the development of your child. Until now, research has not shown a flat out connection among fibroids and fetal development limitations.

- Breech position:

In the event that your fibroids limit space in the uterus, your child might be breech - base down rather than head down. Utilizing ultrasound and an actual test, we screen the child's situation as you draw nearer to your due date. In the event that your child isn't head down your PCP could suggest cesarean segment (C-area) conveyance.

- Preterm conveyance:

Critical fibroid weight might pressure the uterus, prompting preterm constrictions or untimely crack of films (when your water breaks before 37 weeks) and ensuing conveyance. It is essential to contact your Ob/Gyn assuming that you figure you might be in the process of giving birth or releasing liquid.

# Chapter 24

## How to Treat Uterine

## Fibroids Yourself

## (Traditional treatment)

Food and lifestyle changes are many times the principal game plan to treat uterine fibroids. Normal cures, stress the executives, and elective relief from discomfort may likewise assist with facilitating side effects.

Raising vitamin D serum levels might assist with lessening the gamble of fibroids. Notwithstanding, further investigations and exploration that incorporate greater variety are required.

Adjusting pulse

A Dutch report found that there might be a connection between hypertension and fibroids. To deal with your circulatory strain and assist with diminishing your gamble and work on your general wellbeing:

Limit red meat, salt, and added sugar

Check your pulse consistently with an at-home circulatory strain screen

Visit your PCP for ordinary check-ups

talk about pulse readings with your doctor,get standard active work take remedy pulse prescription precisely as endorsed

- Diet and way of life procedures:

Weight reduction. Getting thinner might help forestall or diminish the size of fibroids.

- Nourishment

Your everyday eating routine is a vital consideration for treating fibroids. Eating a nutritious eating regimen can assist you with keeping a moderate weight and decrease your gamble. Certain food sources can likewise assist with facilitating side effects.

# Chapter 25

## Foods To Avoid

As indicated by clinical examinations, eating an abundance of refined starches and food sources with added sugar might set off or deteriorate fibroids. These food sources raise glucose levels, which might make your body produce an excessive amount of insulin chemicals. Limit basic refined sugars like:

White rice, pasta, and flour
Pop and other sweet beverages
Corn syrup
Boxed cereals
Heated products like cakes, treats, doughnuts,chips and saltines.

Furthermore, restricting food sources with added salt, especially handled and bundled foods might be useful. While sodium is a fundamental mineral for wellbeing, the suggested sum for grown-ups is under 2,300 milligrams (about a teaspoon of salt) each day to assist balance with high blood pressure.

# Chapter 26

## Foods To Eat

Fiber-rich natural and entire food sources help:
Increment satiety
Balance chemicals
Forestall overabundance weight gain
Products of the soil additionally assist with lessening aggravation
and lower your gamble for fibroids.

Add these entire food sources to your everyday eating regimen:
Crude and cooked vegetables and natural product
Dried natural product
Entire grains
Earthy colored rice
Lentils and beans
Entire grain bread and pasta
quinoa.

New and dried spices
Milk and dairy might assist with decreasing fibroids. Dairy items
contain high measures of calcium, magnesium, and phosphorus.
These supplements might assist with forestalling the development of
fibroids.

# Conclusion

Medical procedures can frequently assuage torment, weighty dying, and other awkward side effects of uterine fibroids. These techniques can make side impacts. Furthermore, in the event that you have a hysterectomy, you'll at this point not have the option to have kids. Talk with your PCP about pretty much all of your treatment choices. Gain proficiency with the advantages and dangers of every one preceding pursuing your choice. Also,normal treatment of fibroids. Fibroids regularly develop gradually or not by any stretch. As a rule, they recoil all alone, particularly after menopause. You may not require treatment except if you're irritated by side effects. Your PCP will suggest the best treatment plan. You might require a mix of treatments.
In moderate to extreme situations where side effects are troublesome, deteriorating, or not improved with prescription, fibroids might be treated with a medical procedure or ultrasound treatment. Medical procedures might include eliminating only the fibroids or your whole uterus.

At-home consideration, diet changes, and normal cures might assist with treating fibroids and ease side effects. The way of life changes underneath are additionally significant in the counteraction of fibroids.
These normal medicines might possibly help your fibroid side effects, since alleviation really relies on how extreme your side effects are and the way in which your fibroids have advanced. Chat with your primary care physician prior to attempting any of these choices.
Nutrients and Enhancements
Rest
Emotional wellness
Sustenance
At-Home Testing
CBD

Men's Wellbeing
Ladies' Wellbeing.

Medical procedures can frequently assuage torment, weighty dying, and other awkward side effects of uterine fibroids. These techniques can make side impacts. Furthermore, in the event that you have a hysterectomy, you'll at this point not have the option to have kids.

Talk with your PCP about pretty much all of your treatment choices. Gain proficiency with the advantages and dangers of every one preceding pursuing your choice.